The Diary of a Cancer Survivor's Daughter

The Diary of a Cancer Survivor's Daughter

Rebecca J. Bany

iUniverse, Inc.

New York Lincoln Shanghai

The Diary of a Cancer Survivor's Daughter

iUniverse books may be ordered through booksellers or by contacting:

iUniverse
2021 Pine Lake Road, Suite 100
Lincoln, NE 68512
www.iuniverse.com
1-800-Authors (1-800-288-4677)

ISBN-13: 978-0-595-36527-2 (pbk)
ISBN-13: 978-0-595-80961-5 (ebk)
ISBN-10: 0-595-36527-2 (pbk)
ISBN-10: 0-595-80961-8 (ebk)

Printed in the United States of America

This book is dedicated to my mom. The most beautiful, courageous woman I know! I love you mom! Xob

Contents

Introduction

My mom was born on Christmas Eve in the year 1950. She's the baby of her family. She had an older sister and an older brother. Her sister was born with down syndrome. They grew up in a happy home with two loving parents. She grew into a beautiful young woman and became a wonderful mother.

Our home life wasn't always perfect. We had our share of the typical family problems. But for the most part we had a happy life. My childhood memories are fun reminders of my past. My parents struggled to support 5 kids. They did a great job. We never went without. They did their very best to make sure we got everything we wanted.

I remember when we would find something we really wanted, mom would make sure we got it for Christmas or our birthday. They may not have been able to run out and buy it as soon as we asked. But they made sure we eventually got it in the form of a gift. I always wondered if my mom carried a pen and paper in her purse to write down those special items we really wanted. I couldn't figure out how she could always remember exactly what we wanted. Each Christmas was so exciting for me. I knew whatever I had been asking for all year would be under that tree.

Some of us live long lives. Some of us live short lives. But regardless of the length, we live and we learn with each passing day. We are given obstacles. Some we can overcome, others we cannot. I have learned from my mom to live each day to the fullest. She taught me to look at my life, my family, and my friends with eternal love and appreciation.

Introduction

1

It's not cancer

This story is about my mom. She is an incredibly strong woman. She beat cancer. She made it through a long trying ordeal. She is a stronger person because of it, always making the best of a bad situation. She never let it take over. She won.

Although some stories about cancer are written by the individuals who survived the disease itself, it is important to realize that other family members are deeply involved in the experience and survival process as a whole. Family members share in the details of the medical procedures, the fears and anxieties, and the doubts, and so they are affected in their own way. This is my story of my mom's survival.

At the time of my mom's first biopsy, I was very young, only about 20 years old. I hadn't been away from my parents' home for very long. She called me and said, "I just wanted you to know they found a lump in my breast and have to do a biopsy. I don't want you to worry. I'm sure it's nothing." I calmly told her, "Call me as soon as you know something." But when I hung up the phone I cried. I didn't feel like I could talk to anyone about it. I just felt they wouldn't understand why I was so sad when we didn't even know what it was yet. I just curled in a ball on my bathroom floor and prayed for my mom. I didn't think it would be cancer because I just knew that could never happen to my mom.

I wish I had told her I loved her before hanging up the phone. I wish I had reassured her that everything was going to be ok. I felt like she needed me to say that. She needed my hope and faith. I didn't remember the last time I had told her I loved her. It wasn't a big thing in our family. None of us ever told each other we loved one another on a regular basis. It just wasn't a common thing for us. In our family communication wasn't something we did well. We didn't discuss problems or fears. We held it all in and hoped it would go away. Despite our family's reluctance to use words to communicate our emotions, we are a close family. I have the utmost respect and appreciation for my parents.

1

I remember one time I told my brother, Robert, I loved him before we hung up the phone. He said, "Becky don't be stupid." I know he wasn't being ugly. I know he loves me. I just think it was weird for him because we didn't do that in our family. I told my other brother I loved him for the first time I could remember at the funeral of one of his best friends. He told me he loved me too. One of my sisters, April, wrote me a letter when she moved out and told me she loved me and would always be there for me. My other sister, Angi, I never remember saying "I love you" to her or hearing it from her. I feel very bad for that, I want to change it. But I don't know where to start. Actually, I do know where to start; I need to say it to her. If I would just say it that would be a start. I know she would simply tell me she loves me too. I'm afraid of the unknown. It's weird because we all know we love each other. Why is it so hard to say it? I was finally able to say "I love you" to my mother after the biopsy results were shared with the family.

They did my Mom's biopsy a couple days after the initial appointment telling her there was a lump. We had to wait another week before finding out the results. It doesn't sound like a long time. But when you are waiting for results like this, it feels like forever. With each passing day you think about what might happen and how you will handle the results. You try to remain positive. However, you can't help but picture the worst in your mind. Your concerns grow stronger and the thought of losing someone you love weighs heavily on your mind. The results from my mom's biopsy showed she did not have cancer. I was so happy and relieved. But I was still sad too because she had to go through a biopsy. I know cancer is worse. However, I didn't want to see my mom go through any pain. I couldn't bear the thought of her hurting in any way. She is my mom. My own personal super-hero! In my eyes she was Barbie, superman and the incredible hulk all in one.

2

This time it's cancer

I think I took for granted the biopsy was far behind us. Even though I knew lumps could come up at any time and my mom has regular check ups, I didn't expect her to ever have to get another one done. She never misses her yearly exam. There was no way she would get cancer or even another lump. I never wanted to live through that dreadful waiting period for results again. I never wanted her to go through any of it again. Waiting for my mom's results were difficult and stressful. It was one of the hardest things I've ever had to deal with. I'm sure it all sounds selfish that I didn't want to go through it again. I know it was so much harder on her. I can't even imagine the thoughts and dreams she must have had waiting. I worried about her so much. I worried she couldn't take it. I never knew my mom to be sick. I didn't know if she could handle a battle of that degree.

About 5 or 6 years later when my mom told me she would be having another biopsy she sounded very optimistic again. She said, "I've done this before so I'm not really worried about it. Everything will be ok." But in my heart I knew it was cancer this time. I think we all did. I remember my brother telling me he really thought it was going to be cancer because they found more than one lump. I was so scared for her. I tried to convince myself that there was no way she could have cancer. This couldn't happen to my mom. The waiting was horrible. It felt like it took months for the results to come back. At the time I wanted the results back ASAP. I wish I wouldn't have rushed it in my head. I would rather have had no news at all.

A week after the biopsy was done my parents called with the results. I will never forget the day my dad called and tried to make small talk with me. I knew his nervous jokes. I knew his nervous laugh. He was trying to make me laugh before telling me my mom had cancer. I stopped him and said, "Well, what did they say." He said, "Well, it is cancer. But they can get it. She's going to be fine. I just wanted to call everyone so she didn't have to do it." I wanted so much to be strong. I wanted to have courage, but I couldn't. I just broke down. My 14 yr old stepdaughter Kortney was standing behind me. I was still holding the phone to my ear while she was hugging me. I didn't have to tell her anything, she knew. She cried with me and held me for a long time. I felt so bad for my dad. I wish I had been stronger. It was so hard for him to tell me. He immediately called my husband Joe to have him call and check on me.

All I could think about was my mom and all the horror stories I had heard about cancer. I couldn't lose my mom. I didn't want my mom to go through this. I wanted so badly for it to be someone else. I guess I saw my mom as fragile, maybe in my eyes it's because she's my mom and after all those years of protecting me I feel like it's my turn to protect her. Only there was nothing anyone could do for her. We couldn't protect her. She didn't deserve this. Why in the world was this happening to my mom? She had never done anything wrong. I was so mad at God for allowing my mom to get cancer. It was horrible, but I couldn't understand why we have murderers in prison living a healthy life while good people like my mom might not have the opportunity to keep living. I didn't understand and I didn't want it to be my mom. I just couldn't understand why cancer chose her. The reality was my mom, an honest, hard-working woman and mother, has cancer.

Kortney was still crying and I realized right then that she couldn't see me like that anymore. If she saw me that upset she would think I had no hope and I knew she couldn't handle that. She loves her Granny so much. I married Kortney's dad only 3 years ago. She hasn't had enough time with her Granny, it's not fair. So I straightened my face, wiped my tears and told her Granny was going to be just fine. I told her Granny was the strongest lady alive. She was going to beat this. I reassured her many times and got her calmed. I wish I hadn't broken down in front of her. I know that was hard for her to deal with. I know she must have been wishing her daddy had been there. It was too much for anyone, much less a child to take in.

For days all I could think about was my mom and cancer. It was hard for me to believe. I think I was trying to convince myself it wasn't true. I kept thinking the doctor would call her up and say, "Oops, it wasn't cancer after all." Or maybe I was hoping for a miracle, hoping it would just go away. I prayed so hard every night. I asked God to give my mom her own personal guardian angel. I told God I was sorry I was so mad at him. I told God that my younger daughter, my one-year-old Rylee, needed to know her Granny. Rylee needed to have happy memories of Granny.

I begged God to please let mom get through this with as little pain as possible. I worried about her and the pain of cancer. There was so much I didn't understand. But I started reading and I used the internet to research cancer. I didn't want my mom to go through chemo and being sick. I didn't want her to have any pain at all. I wanted her to go in and get a pill or something and the cancer be gone. But deep down I knew it wasn't that easy. Then it hit me hard that my mom was going to lose her hair and possibly lose a breast. I knew these things were superficial and should be the last of everyone's worries. However, my mom was going to go through all of these, every little step. So I couldn't put any of it aside. I needed to go through all of it in my head. I wondered what my mom was thinking about before she went to bed every night. Did she think about this every moment of everyday? My thoughts were consumed by it.

I began looking at Kortney, Rylee and Joe and thanking God for them. I couldn't imagine having to go through the hell my mom was facing. I couldn't imagine them going through what I and my siblings were going through. I never ever want Joe to have to go through what my Dad is going through. Some days it appeared he was getting worse than my mom. He must have been scared out of his mind. My mom is his whole world. She worries about him and thinks about him and has always put him first before anything in her life. Now his life partner was about to experience a hell like no other. She was going to need him more than he could ever imagine. The thought of losing her wore him down so much. You could see it in his eyes and face. But he put on a strong front.

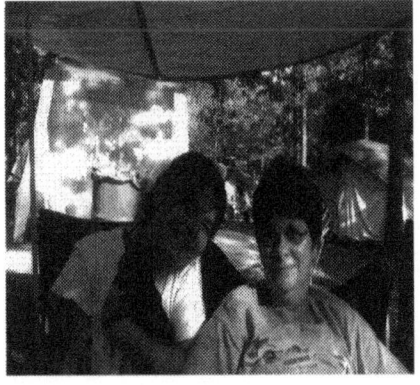

Watching my Dad go through this hardship with my mother got me to thinking about my own family, especially my husband, Joe. There are so many kinds of cancer, and I was worried about Joe getting cancer from chewing tobacco. I beg him every day to quit. I try to explain to him that I can't go through what my dad is going through. What if he's not as lucky and they can't get rid of his. I don't want my husband to ever get cancer. I want him to live forever, with me, but he won't stop. I don't think he understands how much this hurts me or how much it scares me. I don't want Rylee and Kortney to have to watch him go through something like that. I don't know how to get it through to him. I love him so much. This man is my other half and his health means the world to me. I'm so scared for him. I know he won't get breast cancer from dipping tobacco. However, all cancer is bad, no matter where it is. I want my husband to look at me and our children and think about how much he loves us and cares about us. I want that to be enough for him to stop the dipping. I want my love to be all he needs. I've never been able to understand the addiction to anything because I've never had an addiction. So being sympathetic when it comes to that sort of thing is not my best quality.

Joe and I discussed with Kortney what we want to happen when we die. Joe wants to be cremated. I never put a great deal of thought into it. I just always assumed I'd be buried. But if Joe is cremated, I want to be cremated too. I would like our ashes to be combined so that we could be together forever, even in death. Death scares me. The whole idea of death makes me shiver. It makes me sad and full of questions that no one will ever really be able to answer for me. I have faith in my mom. But cancer has never hit so close to me before. It's made me think about my own future and the future of my husband and kids. I find myself looking at life in a different way. I wonder sometimes "Who will be next?"

Thinking about death reminds me of the sudden way my grandfather died. It all makes me remember the day I was at work at the daycare when the director had someone come and pick me up from a field trip with the kids. When I got back to the center she asked me to come into her office. I wasn't sure what was going on. I thought I must have done something wrong. She looked at me very gentle and very sad. She took my hands and said, "Becky, your grandfather was in a car accident." It didn't really phase me. I said, "Well is he ok?" She sat quietly for a second then shook her head no and told me he didn't make it. Until that day I had always prided myself on being strong and not crying in front of other people. I didn't feel it was necessary. But I couldn't control it. I was crushed. I loved him. All those guilt feelings came rushing in. All the time I could have spent with him. I had taken him for granted. I never thought he would die. Then the biggest hurt of all hit, my mom had lost her daddy. My biggest concern was my mom. She was so close to her dad. She loved him so much. I remember at his funeral crying, not only for him, but for her too. I cried because she was going through an enormous amount of pain. I cried because my mom had just lost her father. She would never have him in her life again. I cried for my mom and for her loss.

3

Doctors, doctors, doctors

A week after the second biopsy, my mom had so many doctors visits, so much to take in. She was constantly getting more and more information. Sometimes she had to be there at 7am for an appointment and she would be there the entire day with many other appointments. There was so much she had to know and do and so many rules for her to follow. She couldn't gain or lose weight, she had to watch what she ate, including no caffeine. She had to minimize her time outside the home, making sure she was never with large crowds. And she couldn't exert herself in anyway that would cause her to perspire.

All the time, I was hoping she would remember everything, and especially she was not alone. Of course you see, that's not true either, she was the one with cancer, no one could go through it for her. I knew she wasn't actually alone because other people get cancer. But for me I saw it as only my mom. Sometimes I thought it may be selfish of me to realize there are so many other people out there with cancer and my only concern was my mom. But I couldn't help it. I felt like she needed all of my hope and prayers.

Around this time, I started buying everything I could find with the pink ribbon on it. Then I thought maybe I should be buying stuff that goes to cancer awareness in general. Maybe I shouldn't single one group out. But at the moment I really wanted them to help my mom and get my mom better and find a cure for this and all cancer. I still buy overwhelming amounts of pink ribbon products. Somehow I feel it's my contribution to my mom. I feel like I'm doing this in her honor. I don't do any volunteer work and I know I should. It just makes me feel better to do something and this is my way of helping.

I wondered if she got tired of everyone calling constantly to check on her. I wondered if she just wanted everyone to treat her like nothing was happening. She had so many different tests she had to endure. She even had to get the biopsy done again. One time she told me she wasn't sure if she could go through another biopsy. I cried silently on the phone when she told me they would be doing another one. She said once she was diagnosed and had to go to a specialist, the specialist would be doing another biopsy. I guess it was in order to make his own observations. It wasn't fair. I kept thinking she couldn't take all of this. But she kept saying she would be fine.

I only live 40 minutes away from my mom. But when your mom has cancer 40 minutes feels like forever away. I wanted to be able to be at her house every-day. I wanted to have lunch with her everyday. I wanted to be able to take care of her. I was jealous of my siblings that lived near her because they got to help her more. I wondered if she thought I was a bad daughter. But somewhere inside of me I thought I could pretend it wasn't real, like it wasn't happening, and not liv-ing right next door made it easier to pretend.

They had to put a port on my mom. It's where they hook up the IV line each time for her chemotherapy drip. When she described it to me, I kept imagining a big square hole in her chest where the port would be. I was very nervous about seeing it. But it was nothing like I imagined. It was a small tube coming out of a very small spot on her chest. It wasn't anything like I had pictured. It made me feel better. She said it didn't hurt at all.

My sister took classes and learned to take care of my mom during the chemo. She learned to clean the area where the chemo port was on my mom's chest. I watched her do it once. She had to change gloves and wash her hands many times and be very careful.

I wished I could do it. But that might make it too real for me. I was being self-ish. I didn't want to deal with it. I felt like I was a horrible daughter. All I could do was call and send emails and send pictures that Rylee had colored. I felt like a failure to her. My sisters and sister in law were cooking for my parents every night. I couldn't even help out when it came to that. It's a known fact that I'm no Betty Crocker. I can pick up a bucket of chicken for them. But I can't fry it myself.

My mom needed me for the first time in her life. After all she had done for me over the years, and all I could do was call or email. I was so afraid. I thought if I was there then she wouldn't want me to see her sick. And deep inside I didn't want to see her sick. I wanted to believe she was not sick and in no pain. I was blind and I wanted to be.

I hope someday my mom can understand that I never meant to be a bad daughter to her. I know I owe her everything for simply giving birth to me. I wanted to give her the world and I wanted to take her cancer away. I wanted to close my eyes and for this nightmare to be over. I wanted to twitch my nose and work magic. I didn't believe in magic, I believed in my mom and her ability to beat this. I just couldn't help but think it was too much pain for her, maybe it was too much for me.

4

Chemotherapy

They started the Chemotherapy almost immediately after the second biopsy, approximately one week. Her chemotherapy treatment would be on Friday. Then she would take her medicine for two weeks. Then she would have a week off before starting over. This would be her routine for the next 6 months. This was her cancer prescription as I called it. This was her life, at least during that time.

Each Friday she had chemo I called as soon as it was over and she told me she was fine. Then a couple of days later she started getting really tired really fast. She said she could handle being tired, she was just grateful she wasn't sick. But she looked so sad when she was tired. The chemo just wore her down so much. But no matter how many times I asked her how she was feeling she always had the same answer, "I feel fine. Just a little tired. But nothing I can't handle. I'm just glad I'm not sick." I admired her for being so strong. It sounds really odd, but she made it look easy. I know there is nothing easy about cancer and I know she wasn't always being totally honest with me. But she made me feel better and not so scared for her. I guess she knew exactly what to say and do. I guess that is a Mom's job. She was protecting me and I was grateful for that. I think she knew I was trying to pretend it wasn't real and somehow I don't think she minded.

The whole chemo process seemed to be flying by…. well for me anyways. I can't speak for my mom. I'm sure it wasn't quite the same for her. I looked at it and thought, "oh my gosh, it's almost over. She is doing so well. How is she doing it?" How is she making it through this? No matter how many times she told me it was just a bump in the road, I still doubted that bump. It felt more like an explosion. I think her optimism is what has made this process easier for her. I hear these horror stories about cancer and I know for some people it is exactly that.

Maybe my Mom's was a horror story and she just hid it better than most. I don't know. She's never been one to complain and admit sickness or defeat. My sister told me once that maybe it was worse than my mom let on. This news felt like a car crashing into my heart. What if this was true? Would my mom really hide it if she thought that she was dying?

In my heart I knew she wouldn't hide a fact so important as dying. If she really felt like she wasn't going to make it, she would tell us. I remember one time quite a while ago when she was telling me about her will and how she and dad were getting it in order. I was young at the time. But I remember thinking, "Is she telling me this because something is wrong?" Nothing ever came of it. I didn't think my mom would let us get that kind of surprise. I thought she would prepare us.

During her chemo treatment period, I went to my parent's house with my sister one day to help clean up and mow the lawn. My parents were gone to chemotherapy at the time. While we were there, they got home. My mom went straight in and lay down. I wanted to go in and check on her. Dad came out and told us thanks for everything. He said she was tired and going to take a nap. He really looked like he could use a nap too. I asked him if he was ok. He said, "I'm fine. It's your mom having to go through this." He was so worried about her. He looked as though he had lost weight. He told us he could mow the grass. But I continued to pick up branches and anything else that might affect the lawn mower. My sister continued to mow. I left when Rylee started getting fussy. I knew she was hot and tired from being outside. She was only a year old. But I didn't want to take her inside and wake up my mom.

As the chemotherapy treatments continued, I began to see a puffiness in her face and she looked pale. But still she said she was fine, just tired. Usually, we had our Thanksgiving dinner with mom and dad on the day after the official day so everyone could go to their other family's houses. But we wanted to be with mom on Thanksgiving Day this year because we had so much to be thankful for. However, she insisted and so we went to the home of Joe's mom. The next day we went to my mom's and had a wonderful Thanksgiving dinner and she wasn't sick at all. It was like nothing was wrong with her. We all cooked different dishes and brought them with us so she wouldn't have to do anything. We wanted to show her our appreciation for the many Thanksgivings she had given us. I think we all felt we had taken for granted in the past that mom took care of everything on the holidays. We arrived to a fully cooked holiday meal, not thinking about the time mom had put into making it special for us. I thought this might be something we would continue to do in the future.

5

Chemo on her birthday

I was doing my schedule one day at the beginning of December when I realized my Mom's next chemotherapy would be on her birthday, December 24, Christmas Eve. I was so saddened by this. I didn't want my mom to have chemotherapy on her birthday. I wanted her to have a normal birthday. She'd been having bad birthdays for a couple of years. In 1999 on her birthday, Christmas Eve, she found her mom dead. It was horrible. She and her sister had gone to visit. My mom asked me to go with them. But I didn't feel like going all the way out to Granny's house, so I stayed behind. It was so far away, and well it was my Granny's house, she was so old. I was so guilt stricken for not going with her, but I just couldn't bring myself to do it. To this day I feel horrible for not going. I wish I could have been the one to open that door and find Granny. I would have done anything to shield her from that. What kind of God lets my mom find her mother dead on her birthday? How horrible is it that for the rest of my mom's life on her birthday she would have that image? I wanted to steal it from her.

Other difficult and sad things had happened to my mom during holidays. My grandpa died in a car accident only 10 months after my Granny died. That made her holidays sad too. She no longer had a mother or father. All she had was her sister. I felt like luck just wasn't on her side. When I was very young my mom's brother died of cancer. I couldn't understand why all of these bad things were happening to her. I was sad that my grandparents had died and I felt guilty for not spending time with them. But the majority of my grief was out of fear and sadness for my mom. She was hurting and there was nothing anyone can do to help her.

My mom said she decided to do her chemotherapy on Christmas Eve, her birthday, because she didn't want to get off of her schedule. Plus, we were having Christmas at her house on Christmas Day. She said she wouldn't be doing anything that day anyway. But the thought of it was still horrifying. Would she be thinking about it being her birthday and yet she was having a chemotherapy drip instead of a birthday cake? I know those nurses have lots of patients, but do you think maybe one of them could remember to tell her happy birthday. I'm sure it's too much to ask. But it would be nice.

Although having chemotherapy treatment the day before was not a very nice way to celebrate mom's birthday, the following day, Christmas day, was beautiful. Our whole family had a big group picture taken. We haven't had family pictures taken since I was in high school. My mom had commented several times that she would like a group picture of the grand kids. So we had their picture taken too. When she and my dad opened it I was video taping. She cried the sweetest cry. She was so happy. I think it even touched my dads heart. You could see emotion in his eyes. He too loved the picture. We had steak and shrimp this Christmas instead of turkey and dressing like normal. Everyone loved it. Instead of drawing names for Christmas this year we played a game, some call it white elephant. We had so much fun. It was so nice to see the family sit together and laugh. On every family occasion, my sister brings deviled eggs. My brother loves her deviled eggs. This time she showed up with the outside of the deviled eggs. She had forgotten the filling. We laughed at her all day. She may never live it down.

After Christmas mom got sick and they had to put her on antibiotics. I was scared for her because all I had heard the whole time was how bad it is for a cancer patient to catch something. Someone mentioned maybe she got it at Christmas when we were all there. I suddenly thought, "maybe it's my fault because Rylee had been sick before Christmas." My daughter had no fever on Christmas Day and appeared to be fine. But what if she wasn't and that is why mom got sick. I felt horrible. I felt like everyone in the family was thinking how rotten it was for me to be so insensitive. Then I was told that she had started getting sick before we were there on Christmas. Mom said her antibiotics worked well and fast. She wasn't sick long. That was a relief. I was worried that maybe it would take so much longer because of the chemotherapy damaging her immune system.

Over the following six weeks, I called my sister a lot to ask how mom felt. I didn't want to bombard mom with phone calls, especially if she didn't feel well. Then a realization hit me, what if this chemotherapy didn't work. Was that a possibility? Was there a chance that she was going through all of this and would die anyway? I began to get very upset and overwhelmed with these thoughts. I asked my sister in law. She said that she was under the impression that mom's doctors really felt like they could get all of the cancer out. They seemed to be very positive about her beating this. My mom had done so well during this whole ordeal. She followed the doctor's orders to the very last period. I'm very proud of her. Not everyone has the strength and will power she does. Not everyone could remain so upbeat about cancer.

6

The "C" word

Cancer.... the word is disgusting to me. It makes me mad. It makes me sad. It makes me angry. It makes me scared. I don't understand it. I don't understand why there even has to be cancer. I don't understand why there is no easier way, why there is no cure. Sometimes I can't even describe how that word makes me feel. I'm afraid of getting cancer myself. Now when I get a pap smear I am terrified of the "C" word. I am a nervous wreck awaiting those results. It seems like it takes forever for them to arrive in the mail. Then I get that relief when I read the words "negative." But I can't help but wonder will I always get that negative. My sister in law tells me they won't do mammograms until I turn 35. I think that is ridiculous. Why not do them from the time we start pap smears? Wouldn't it be safer and save more lives? Anytime I ask people those questions they say I don't know. My mom has breast cancer. I want a mammogram every year even though I'm only 27.

I just read a book about a woman who got breast cancer at 27 years old. The book was so helpful. The author made me realize a lot of the things my mom is going through. My mom would never tell me those things. Reading that book gave me a different outlook. I felt so sad for that woman through the entire book. I cried while I read it. I opened it and did not put it down that day until I had finished reading the entire book. This woman lived through hell and made it. She was so strong and so positive. She treated it like what it was, a horrible disease, but a horrible disease that could be beaten.

I wanted to give the book to my mom to read. But I didn't want to overstep my bounds. What if she didn't want to read a book about cancer? I just think maybe she would think it was inconsiderate of me to force a cancer book on to her. Kind of like how I feel when other people tell me about their mom's cancer story and how it was this way or that way for them. I think to myself, but this is my mom. It's completely different because it's my mom. I know that sounds selfish. But I can't think about anyone else except my mom. She always eats right and plays by the book and exercises and she has cancer. Even the sentence doesn't sound right.

I love my mom so much. I know I don't always agree with everything she agrees with. Our thinking isn't always the same. But that doesn't change the fact that I think she's a queen. I may not agree with everything, but I don't think she is wrong either.

I love my children very much. I have many parenting techniques that differ from those of my moms. I think that's part of the glory of parenting and having children. You teach morals and values and you do the very best you can possibly do to raise them right. And even though they don't make every choice the same as you doesn't mean you can't still be proud of them. It's part of a changing world and individuality. We all do things that we hope our children can correct in their lives and do better. We always want better for our children.

I know my mom feels that way about us. She never criticizes how I raise my kids. She even knows how to give those perfect answers when I ask her for parenting advice. She doesn't give me a definite answer. She gives one of those answers that makes me figure out what I think is best for my children. And what I think is best may not have been what was best for me when I was a kid. But my mom understands that.

You hear so much about these horrible moms that let bad things happen to their children or that just neglect them. You hear about these moms that just don't seem to care. But I will never understand how that is possible. I love my girls more than I can ever imagine loving. It's an overwhelming love. It's the most powerful kind of love there is. I know my mom feels that way about each of her children too. I can feel it. I hope my children can feel it too.

My mom had her last chemo treatment in January 2005. I was so happy. She said this was the worse dose of all the chemo treatments she's had. She got the most sick and tired with this one. It seemed to take longer for her to recover from this one. My mom had been doing chemotherapy for 6 months and still working at her full-time job as a payroll secretary. I told you she could be Superwoman's sister. At first I was thinking, "thank goodness, it's over, then I realized, it's not over. Now she has to do surgery to have her mastectomy. Then she will do her radiation. Then if she chooses she will have reconstructive surgery. She still has a long road ahead of her. But as long as that road is leading her to get better, I guess it's a good road.

My mom tells us her cancer was caused by the estrogen in her menopause meds. I am so mad that no one told her they could cause cancer. I'm so mad they didn't test my mom to find out if those meds could give her cancer. Why didn't they? I want to scream at the doctor that told her to take those meds for menopause. All of this could have prevented if they would have just told this information ahead of time. It should be mandatory that this information be given and the proper test should be ran. Her doctor said that none of them women in her bloodline should take anything with estrogen in it. My mom said menopause is hard, but we have to tough it out. I know she wishes someone had told her that too.

7

Preparing for the future...

When I found out my mom had cancer, I sat down and went over my will making sure it was up to date. I made sure we have plenty of life insurance policies just in case. I wrote a letter to Joe, one to Kortney and one to Rylee. I put them in the burn box in the event that something happens to me. If ever I'm told I have cancer I want to be somewhat ready for it. I know you can never really be ready. But I think it may help to have my affairs in order. I want my family to always know how much I love them. I want them to be able to see it in my words instead of just hearing it from other people. I think it would mean more that way. I write every little thing down in their lives just in case I'm not here to tell them about it one-day. I stress to my girls not to ever take anything with estrogen in it. I told them it's always better to be safe than sorry and we are all tougher than we think. Find the strength inside!

My sister called me one day and said that my mom didn't think she was going to have the reconstructive surgery after the mastectomy. She said mom had found out that when she gained or lost weight that the reconstructed breast would not gain and lose with her. But her other breast would. I wondered if really she was just scared of the cancer coming back again and would feel safer without the breast. I respect any decision she makes. It doesn't make a difference to me how many breasts she has, just as long as she's alive!

I read about a woman who chose to have a full mastectomy done, even though she didn't actually have breast cancer herself, but rather because her mom and grandma had died of breast cancer. It seemed like a good idea. But I wondered how old she was. It seemed like a huge decision. I couldn't say I wouldn't make the same decision. It sounds very scary. In my head I think, no way would I do that. No way would I just let someone take my breast. But in my heart I think about all the suffering that would be prevented. I don't want my children to go through the fears and sorrows of having a mother with breast cancer. I think it takes a very mature person to make a decision of that capacity. Maybe I'm not that mature yet. Or maybe since I haven't gone through what she's gone through it's something I can't understand in the way she can. But I do have to say that woman had a tremendous amount of courage and love for herself and others to do all she has done. I admired her.

On a Friday night we were going out to dinner because my mom would have her mastectomy on the following Tuesday. Our dinner went well. We ate at a Mexican restaurant. It was good food. Mom and Dad seemed so tired. They had a day full of doctor's visits, exams and paperwork. You could definitely tell it was in the back of everyone's mind. Maybe it helped that we were all together and there for one another. We, myself, Robert, Angi, April, Michael and all of our families were with our parents trying to organize all of the details ahead of time. It was weird because we were all out to dinner, but it wasn't a celebration. I guess it could have been called a celebration because she had completed the chemother-apy so heroically. But really it was a way for us to say we'd all be with her in prayer while she was in surgery. We would all love her no matter what.

My mom had a worried look on her face, as she should. After all, she was the one who was going under the knife. I guess that was probably the only thing she could think about right then. She kept busy. But I know it had to linger around her constantly. I wasn't the one having surgery and I couldn't stop thinking about it. The closer it got, the more my stomach turned.

I wanted to take Rylee and Kortney to the hospital with me when mom had surgery. I didn't want to leave Rylee with a babysitter. I felt like she needed me. I know she would have been fine with the sitter. I know Kortney had to go to school. She didn't need to be stressing in a hospital all day. But something in me kept saying that I shouldn't leave either of them on a day like that. Maybe they wouldn't need me as much as I would need them. I guess I was so scared for my mom that I was having a hard time of leaving my babies.

I had been trying to explain to Joe that instead of leaving Rylee with the sitter that day I would rather have had him stay with her. But he said he had to work. I don't think he gets it. I don't expect him to get it though. He's never been through this. Plus, if I don't understand it myself, how can I expect him to understand it. Kortney asked me if I thought Granny would one day let her see where they took the breast from. I told her probably so. She asked me if it was weird for her to want to see. But I told her it really wasn't. It was normal. Maybe it was something Kortney needed to see to help her learn and understand about cancer and how serious it is.

On the day before mom's surgery, I wondered if she had slept at all. She would find out between 3pm and 5pm that day what time the surgery would be. It was like a countdown. I didn't know why they couldn't already tell her. Maybe it was just that busy. There's just too much cancer out there. I wanted to call her. I wanted to hold her hand while they told her what time they would be performing the mastectomy on her left breast. I can't imagine her thoughts through this.

I wanted to ramble on and on to whomever would listen until mom called to tell me what time the surgery took place. I just couldn't call her yet. I was afraid she would hear the fear in my voice. I didn't want to cause her anymore stress than what she already had. I wished I could be there to comfort her. But I didn't think I could have really been that comforting to my mom. I try. But I'm not sure I'm good at it. It's hard for me not to cry and beg God not to let hurt come to my mom. She's a beautiful woman and she always will be. I know when something like this happens everyone thinks they have the greatest mom and of course, their mom doesn't deserve this. But it's really true in my mom's case.

8

Mastectomy surgery

Kortney asked me if I was scared for my mom. I told her no, not at all. I told her Granny is a strong lady. But in my head I was freaking out! I couldn't tell her I was scared for my mom. I was afraid she would get worried and stress about it all day instead of concentrating at school. She's too young too worry about these things. The night before my mom's surgery I couldn't sleep at all. I tried so hard. I even tried actually counting sheep! I kept looking at the clock. I just wanted it to be 4am so I could go ahead and get up and get ready to go. My brothers and sisters were picking me up. Mom had to be there at 6am and they would start the surgery around 7am. My mom must have laid there all night thinking about the following morning. I kept thinking to myself, it's a surgery that's done everyday. It's no big deal. Don't worry about it. But there's no way you can not worry when it's your mom. She could be in there for an ingrown toenail and I would worry.

My clock doesn't tick out loud like you see in tv. But I swear I couldn't almost hear it. Then it was 4am. I got up and got dressed. Then I changed clothes. I wasn't sure what I was suppose to wear. First I had on sweat pants and a t-shirt because I knew we would have to wait a while and I wanted to be comfortable. But then I decided to put on a nice pair of jeans and a better shirt. I should at least look a little nice. Why was I worrying about comfort when my mom was going to have someone cutting on her? It was ridiculous and I shouldn't be think-ing of myself right now.

Then it hit me, I was going to see my mom for the first time without her wig. I was so scared. Not because I thought she might look horrible or anything. But because I would have to see her scared and bald and this whole ordeal will be more real. It's so stupid. Even in my head it's stupid. But I don't want to have the image of my mom being the cancer patient like you see on TV. I feel horrible for those people. They are just people that are sick and need extra love and support, just like my mom. But I'm so scared for all of those people. I'm so scared they won't have another day to depend on. I feel bad for what they have to go through. I just don't want to think of my mom like that too. I wanted my mom to still be my mom. I can't really explain it. She's still my mom. It's so hard to put those kind of thoughts into words and make people understand. All morning long I prepared myself and I realized what I was really scared of. I was scared that I would see my mom with no hair and break down. I couldn't do that to my mom. She needs me to be very strong right now.

The ride to the hospital was quiet. Nothing was said about my mom's cancer or surgery. Every now and then my sisters would crack a joke to lighten the mood. But I knew everyone was just as scared as I was. Even though the hospital is only about half an hour from my house, the drive there seemed to take forever.

As soon as we got there they let us go straight back to see her. She had a surgical hat on so you couldn't see that she was bald at all. It made me feel so much better. But man did she look scared. Her face was very red. It was almost like no one knew what to say. We asked her how she felt and if she needed anything. Then a nurse came and told us only my dad could be in there with her at that time. We went to the waiting room and waited for my dad to join us. They said they would be taking her back at 6:30am for the surgery to begin. But at 6:50am we began to get worried because dad still hadn't come to the waiting room. We finally got a hold of him. They forgot to get my mom to sign a consent form so that was the hold up. They had to get her signature.

About 7am my dad came in and we headed to the cafeteria to get breakfast. There were lots people in there. I felt bad for each and every face I looked at because I knew they were there for someone they loved also. I was glad we were all there, not only for mom, but for dad. I can't imagine him having to sit there all by himself with nothing to do but think. In the waiting room we talked and read books and magazines and walked around. A volunteer told us we were on the wrong floor waiting room. We changed waiting rooms and didn't have as good of seats so it was harder for us to chat with one another. The volunteer lady on that floor was very nice and worked hard. She was constantly running around the hospital helping people and talking to them and reassuring them. All of that work and no pay. What a wonderful person.

While waiting we watched a Marti gras parade through the hospital. The children patients with cancer came through and everyone put beads on them. There was music and fun. The kids really seemed to enjoy it. But for me it was so sad for those poor babies. Two of them that came through looked as though they were only about 5months old. I thought of Rylee and Kortney and how much I love them. It made me want to hug them and squeeze them and never let go. It made me so grateful my babies are ok. My sister cried. I knew she must be thinking the same thing about her children. Rylee did end up staying with Joe today. I must have drove them crazy with phone calls to check on her. There was a lady in the lobby playing the piano and one playing the violin. It was beautiful soothing music. I was so amazed that these people volunteered their time just to help others. It gave me a new perspective on volunteer work and the people who do it. They are amazing people with a special place in heaven.

Finally the doctor told us that mom came through it great. He said it looks as though they got it all. But he won't know for sure until the test come back from the lab. That will probably be about 5 days, a long hard time to wait. I was very happy to hear how positive the doctor was. It gave me hope.

The doctor came and told us mom was waking up from the surgery. While she was in recovery we couldn't see her. But the volunteer gave us updates on her. She came out and told us mom wanted her glasses and scarf. She said mom was sitting up reading. But they still didn't have a room available for her. The volunteer said we could go eat lunch and if there was anything else she would come to the cafeteria and get us. Once we got to the cafeteria we saw that it was packed. There were no empty seats. So we got out food to go and sat in the waiting room and ate together. You hear horrible things about hospital food. But this hospital was amazing. The food was actually good.

When the volunteer came back this time she said they had found a room for mom but it would have to be cleaned so we would have to wait a couple more hours before we could see her. So we all chipped in and got mom a big assortment of flowers and plants. We also got her two different cards, one funny, one sentimental. And we put a small glass cross that said mom in with the cards. They told us we could go ahead and wait for her in her room. Once in there we saw she had a dry erase board. We decided to leave her a funny message to make her laugh. My sister wrote "We love you mom, Feliz Navidad, Get Well soon (backwards), git r done, Love your family!." We were in her room for about 40 minutes before they brought her in. We were watching a movie about Patsy Cline. There were no TV's in the waiting room so we were a little happy to have something to take our minds away for a minute! I could tell by the look on my mom's face that she was happy to see all of us there when they wheeled her in. I knew at that moment she felt very loved. My dad was so relieved to see her. He had his strong face on all day. But the way he held her hand when he saw her was like fireworks. He needed to see with his own two eyes that she was ok.

When my dad asked her how she was feeling, she said she wasn't in any pain at all. They had given her morphine at 10:45am. But the doctor was amazed. She said the morphine had worn off by then and if mom needed anything at all to let them know. She told her this is not a time to be tough. Do not try to do this without pain meds. If you need anything just let us know. But the entire time we were there mom said she was fine and in no pain at all. She said she would probably ask for pain meds before bed just in case.

That evening together in her room was a very special experience,we stayed with her for a long time. We made sure she ate dinner. They said she could eat anything she wanted. The only thing she had all day was a graham cracker after the surgery. She was getting hungry!! She was laughing and joking and sitting up in her bed. I couldn't believe this woman just had a breast removed. When the guys left the room she asked us girls if we wanted to see. I was very scared, but also curious. I did want to see. I really thought it might help me understand more about what she is going through. It was nothing as I expected. It wasn't scary looking at all. It was flat like a table with no nipple. There was just a line of stitches across where the breast had been. I hope I never have to go through this. But if I do, I hope I can be as strong and brave as my mom.

I don't understand all of the medical details, but I remember that she had two drainage catheter things to drain the fluids from where the breast was. The doctor said he removed 2 of the 3 lymph nodes. I wasn't even sure what a lymph node was. We watched a video teaching us how to clean where the drain tubes are so she doesn't get an infection. My sister in law and sister would actually get to watch a nurse do it because they would be doing it for my mom when she got home.

It was hard to leave her there in the hospital and go home without her. I wanted to stay with her in case she got scared or in case something unforeseen happened. When we left we gave her a hug and kiss bye and told her we loved her. I didn't want to leave her there. I wanted to take her with us. But I knew she was with my dad and all those doctors and she would be getting out the next day. The way home there was more talking and less tense air. We had been there for our mom and dad when they needed us the most. We had made her day easier in our own way. I watched my sisters little boy the next day while she and my sister in law went back to the hospital to watch the nurse clean the drain tube area. I wanted so badly to go back and sit with mom until they sent her home. But I knew they needed to be there more. I wanted to call that morning. But I know how hard it is to talk on the phone when you have doctors and nurses in and out. So, I decided to wait until she got home. My sister said she still wasn't in any pain, just sore. They had sent my mom home with vicoden just in case. My mom is very hard headed when it comes to pain meds. She will not take them unless it is absolutely necessary. She has always said she does not like the way they make her feel. I know I've said it before, but it's worth saying again, that woman is just too strong!!

It was great to talk to both my mom and my sister about how well things were going. Mom said she felt fine, as always. She was just tired because they didn't get much sleep last night in the hospital. She said it was too loud and the nurses were in there so much checking on her that at 5am they finally just turned the light on. But she said she was very happy to be home. I asked her if she was hurting. She said no. She said she had been doing the exercises they told her to do and they didn't hurt either. I told her how I found bird feathers in the closet the night before. Apparently my cat had been bringing them in and eating them in my closet. I had to keep the door shut from then on. I thought maybe I would tell her that so we didn't only have to talk about cancer. I was sure sometimes she wanted to have a normal conversation again. I was so happy she was ok. I was so happy she was doing so well. I talked to my sister the next morning. She said that mom did so well the night before. She slept through the night with no pain meds. I'm amazed by my mom. I keep telling everyone how well she's doing. I don't even care if they get tired of me babbling on. But everyone in my life seems to genuinely care. It's really great to see how much they care. One of my friends is taking my parents dinner tonight. I can't express how grateful I am to have a friend like that.

9

God didn't let me down

My mom was doing so good. She did her exercises everyday and still had no pain. My sisters and sister in law all live near her so they cleaned the drainage tubes everyday. They said it all looked good. On that Sunday she went to my nieces 17th birthday party. It hadn't even been a week since the surgery. She didn't act any different. If you didn't know, you couldn't tell she had just had a mastectomy surgery. I hope that I have at least half of the strength and courage she has. It boggles my mind how she is always so strong and happy. Through this whole process she didn't let it get her down.

I received an email from a friend. She heard from a lady we used to work with. This lady is one of the nicest ladies you could ever meet. She was always an honest and upbeat lady full of love and happiness. Her husband was diagnosed with cancer and it has spread. Things aren't looking good for him. But she still has hope and faith. I cried as I read the letter. It made me sad that she is now in another state and there's nothing we can do for her. I know we can pray and I hope she feels our prayers. She has her children near and I'm sure they are a big help to her. These are good people, like my mom. It makes me so mad that this is happening to these wonderful people. I know it's nothing they've done because there is nothing they could have done to deserve this pain and heartache. Then would is it? Why are innocent people suffering and dying of cancer? I wonder if these questions will ever be answered. There's so much we don't know. How close are we to a cure?

I found out that her husband passed away. I will keep her and her family in my prayers tonight. I wish he could have made it. It makes me so sad to think that family lost a husband, a father and a grandfather. I also found out another lady I use to work with has cancer. She is such a sweet, wonderful lady. I know she's strong and she will overcome this. But I can't help but think about how hard this is for her and her family. I will keep them in my prayers also. It just feels like cancer has gotten out of control. It seems to be taking over and not so slowly anymore.

Then my mom was awaiting her pathology results to insure the cancer hasn't spread anywhere else and that they got it all. It's all about waiting and wondering. You never know what's next or what tomorrow might bring. I wished I could answer the phone for her when they called. I felt in my heart that the news would be positive. My sister said she expected them to call the next day. The doctor told us after the surgery that he felt positive that they got it all. But he couldn't be certain until the pathology results came back. I hoped the positive feeling I had would turn out to be right.

I was thinking one night that I'd been really upset with God for letting this happen to my mom. It really had me upset. But then I realized I had been asking God to make the cancer go away or at least don't make my mom go through pain. I told him I forgave him for the cancer thing. But asked him to please not make it hard on my mom. "Please don't make her suffer," I prayed. I guess I had taken for granted how strong my mom was. I didn't realize maybe my prayers were working. I thought I wasn't doing anything for my mom. But maybe I was. All of my prayers were being answered. I still wanted my prayer about the cancer diagnosis being wrong to come through for me. But it didn't. However, God listened when I asked him to help my mom get through this. Thank you God. I really appreciate everything. Keep up the good work!

10

Cancer free

My brother prepared me for what results might come back from these pathology tests. He said he read it's common for people to still have cancer even after chemotherapy. But since the hormone therapy given afterwards is so strong, it kills the cancer cells that the chemotherapy missed. I'm glad he told me that. I had no idea and knowing this made me feel like if there was some cancer left, I could take it and my mom could take it. She could take it on and beat it, just like she'd done so far.

My mom got her pathology results back and the doctor said, "she is considered to be cancer free." They told her that they found cancer in the lymph nodes they took out. But they found none in her body. They said if there were any they would be so small that they were undetectable. But with the hormone treatment she was taking it would wipe out anything left. They said the hormone treatment is so much stronger than the chemotherapy. She will take this pill for 5 years.

Mom and I talked about her experiences with cancer and surgery and life during all of this. She wasn't sure when her radiation would start. But she sounded so positive and happy. It was nice to hear my mom really happy again. I told her that watching her go through this and seeing how strong and positive she has been has really helped everyone. I feel like if I ever have to go through this I can do it. When we first found out she had cancer I really felt like I didn't know how she was going to do it. I thought if it ever happened to me then I wouldn't be able to handle it. But seeing my mom run through the cancer process nonstop with a constant smile, it's helped me realize you have to keep a positive outlook! Maybe my mom wasn't always so positive, but she never let on to us, her children, how hard it really was. Mom told me that when they first told her she cried and couldn't figure out how she was going to get through this. She said something just triggered in her head that she doesn't have a choice and she can either make it through or give up. She choose to beat cancer and that's what she has done. She said they told her that having a positive attitude has helped her so much.

My mom said her hair was growing back, very light. I know she meant gray! I had never seen my mom with gray hair. I was sure she'd have it colored as soon as she could. My brother said she got a new wig. He said it looked so good. I planned to go visit on the weekend. I couldn't wait to see it. I couldn't wait to see my mom and how well she was doing. I knew she had to be happy she to be getting her hair back. I didn't know how long it would take to grow back. But I was thinking a couple of months. She didn't like it long so that wouldn't be an issue. After going through all of this, maybe she would dye it pink and grow it to her toes! Hahaha! Just joking mom!!! It's nice to be able to joke again. It's ok to be happy. Thanks again God!

Two weeks after my mom's surgery, she went in and had the tubes taken out. She called me and was so happy. The doctor told her that there was no way the cancer had spread to any other part of her body. He said that the cancer that was in the lymph nodes he took out wasn't on the outside or something along those lines or maybe those lympnods weren't on the outside. Anyways, the point is that it couldn't have spread into the rest of her body. You could hear the happiness in her voice. She said she was supposed to start the radiation sometime in March.

My moms doctor told her diet can make a difference with cancer. She said her doctor said lots of people who get cancer do not eat the correct amount of fruits and vegetables per day or exercise on a regular basis. It really made me think about my own eating habits. I'm doing the Atkins diet right now and it's actually working very well for me. I get plenty of vegetables. But I don't get as much fruit as I should. But it says I can slowly introduce some fruits into my diet. So I'm going to do that. I also plan to start walking a mile or so everyday. I was so good at eating right and walking everyday when I was pregnant. But after I had the baby, I just slacked off so much. But now I feel like it's a matter of life or death. I have to make myself do this. I have to have more will power and just be a stronger healthier person.

Mom went through radiation next. I wondered how that would be. My sister said someone told her it was worse than chemotherapy and that it was horrible. But my brother in laws mom told him that it wasn't so bad. She said it just felt like she had a sunburn all the time. My mom flew through it. She'd soared high through the whole thing so far! I had no doubt that my mom could handle anything. I wasn't so scared about the radiation. Of course, it wasn't me going through it. But I got the impression on the phone that she wasn't real scared of it either. I love my mom. She's an incredible woman. I can't believe she's gone through so much and she's still so happy and positive. She's given me and I'm sure I can speak for my siblings, a great amount of hope and faith about life and the hardships it can throw your way. No matter what life throws at me I now know I can and will win if I just fight and believe.

11

The process

I have been thinking a lot about the process of killing cancer. First there's the chemotherapy, then the mastectomy, then hormone therapy and radiation, last the reconstruction, not to mention all of the healing time. It's called neoadjuvant therapy when you are given chemotherapy, radiation or hormone therapy before the surgery. Its purpose can be for cosmetic reasons or to reduce the size of area in which the surgery will be performed. Doing this can actually shrink the cancer before the surgery. Cancer takes years of your life away, some a little less, some a little more. If I'm hearing it right and the hormone therapy is so much stronger than chemotherapy, then why not do that first, why chemotherapy at all? Or, if they are going to do a mastectomy, why do the chemotherapy and risk it spreading? Why not just do the mastectomy first and get it out right then? I'm so confused, I don't understand. I don't get the chemotherapy process and why it has to be so hard. I know I'm not a doctor and I'm sure there's so much I don't know about cancer. It just seems like there might be an easier way. I guess to fully understand it you have to hold a medical degree and sometimes I wonder if they totally get it. Maybe they just get the medical part, not the whys and how comes.

My mom told me that my sister in laws father came through his surgery and is doing well. She said that she talked to his wife and his spirits are high. She said he may even get out today. I felt so bad when my sister in law found out her dad had cancer. It was right after my mom found out. It must be difficult when you have parents on both sides with cancer, very scary. I'm very happy her father made it through his surgery successfully. Before my mom went through this I never put much thought into cancer and how hard it really is to beat. Now I know there is so much more to beating cancer than merely strength and faith. Even with the best of luck or the most positive attitude, cancer can still win. Sometimes the strongest can't beat cancer. It takes a lot of love and even more belief in yourself to just get through each day. But still there are no guarantees with cancer. I'm very proud of those who have the strength and courage to even take on cancer, whether they beat it or not.

My mom was really returning to her life before cancer in a big way and she looked great. I saw mom's new wig at my nieces birthday party. It looked so awesome. I loved it. It was slightly shorter and darker with a reddish tint. It looked so good on her. It made her look younger. It was amazing how real it looked. The first one looked real too, but this one was even better. I wondered if after her hair grew back she'd miss the wig. She was doing so well since her surgery. She went back to work only 3 weeks after her surgery. I knew she was happy to be back. She didn't like sitting around. She kept herself busy! Plus, I knew she had missed her friends at work. She talked about them a lot. They seemed like great people. She had to love her job. She'd been there for a long time. They must have treated her right. I know they were wonderful throughout this whole process. They were always doing wonderful things for her. I thought about going up there and meeting her for lunch. But I figured she had lots of catching up to do with the people in her office.

It's weird because in my head I keep thinking the whole cancer thing is over. But I know it's not. I mean in a way it is. The cancer is gone, but she still has radiation and reconstruction. I'm not sure if she'll actually do the reconstruction. For some reason I don't think she will. But who could blame her. After going through all of this do you really want to add anything else to it. I totally understand if she doesn't. But who knows, she may surprise me!

12

Radiation

Mom started her radiation. She had wanted to start it after her spring break (she works at the school). But they told her they really didn't want to wait just in case it had spread and they just hadn't caught it. She went every morning (Monday thru Friday) at 8:15am. She said they had her lay on a pillow and put her left arm up and they had a pillow they formed to her body. She used that pillow every time she went. The radiation only went over that area of her body where the cancer was found. She said it made her a little tired in the afternoon and the doctor told her that would get worse. The doctor also said she would get a sunburn from the radiation on that area of her body where the radiation was being performed. But that hadn't happened yet. But he said it probably would in another week or so. She was doing radiation for about 2 weeks. We went camping her first week into radiation. She appeared to be back to normal. You would have never known she was going through radiation for breast cancer. You can't tell that she only has one breast. I was surprised because I thought it would be a major difference. But it really wasn't noticeable.

We had a wonderful Easter. We spent the day at mom's house. I think we all felt after what she has gone through we really needed and wanted to spend the whole day with her. She was very happy. We had BBQ and watched the kids hunt eggs. Everyone seemed to really enjoy themselves. I slacked off on the holidays once I got married. It's hard when you have to share your holidays between families. But this year I wasn't missing anything with my mom, everyone would just have to understand that. The first 2 years after I met my husband I didn't go to my mom for Easter at all. I thought, "it's just Easter." But after she got cancer every holiday seemed more important to me. My mom is always doing Thanksgiving the day after Thanksgiving so that everyone can go to their other families house on Thanksgiving day. Me and my siblings have already told mom we won't be doing that this year. We will definitely have Thanksgiving day at her house on Thanksgiving day this year!

Mom calls me almost every morning on her way to work after radiation. It really nice because we to talk about so much. I feel like we are making up for lost time. I always talked to my mom, but never as much as now. When we talk she always seems very interested and she always asks about the girls. She visits the girls and takes in every minute with them. I found that my mom and I talk about more now. Before it didn't seem as though we talked about our feelings or emotions. But now she is more open with me. She tells me about her thoughts and she is interested in my thoughts. I guess after battling cancer you realize how important it is to soak in every minute with your family because at any minute it can all be gone. I know I've learned that lesson from this whole experience.

Sometimes I feel bad because she is the person that calls me almost everyday. Then I go on and on telling her stories. I have to tell myself, "ok, she's the one with cancer. She doesn't want to hear about you." But sometimes I think she does. I think it makes her feel better to hear about something other than cancer. I sent her flowers when she finished her chemotherapy. She called to tell me thank you and wanted to know what they were for. I told her just because. They really were just because.......... just because she finished chemo, just because she beat cancer, just because she's a survivor, just because I love her so very much, just because I wanted her to smile when she saw how beautiful they were, just because she deserved them.

13

Life

I got an update on how my mom was doing with her recovery recently. Mom came by and spent a few hours with me and Rylee. We went to lunch with Joe. It was really nice. I think she really enjoyed playing with Rylee. She had radiation that morning, then a physical therapy consultation that afternoon. Instead of driving home she came here between appointments. They had to do physical therapy to teach her some things to do to get the blood to flow regularly through her arm and fingers. I don't know if all of my facts are completely accurate. But I'm stating them the best I can remember and understand. They told her they had to do something about her scar also because it was too tight. The doctor said it should have loosened by then. They ripped a piece of tape off of her and skin came off with it. She had to start putting more lotion on the area where they were doing the radiation.

Joe's grandpa came by as well. He asked about my mom. It was so sincere and sweet how he listened to exactly what I had to say. He really cared. Sometimes you think people are just asking because they feel obligated. But it's nice when you run across those people that are so genuine.

I've been thinking lately about people and cancer and putting their lives at risk. I watch people smoke their cigarettes and put dip in their mouth and etc. They know these things cause cancer. My sisters and my husband have watched my mom go through all of this and still they smoke/dip. I wonder how they can't possibly be scared of having to endure the same process. It scares me for them. Now maybe I don't understand because I've never been addicted to anything. But I honestly don't think I will ever understand it. I can't stand it when people say "well you have to die someday" or "you gotta die of something." That is the most idiotic thing I have ever heard. It's crap if you ask me. Why would you want to die sooner and suffer? It makes no sense to me. Plus, why would you want to put your family through that kind of pain on purpose? You know what you are doing can cause you to have cancer and yet you still do it. Why don't people think more of their family and loved ones? I love my mom with all of my heart and I know my siblings do to. I guess that's why it makes it that much harder for me to understand people smoking and dipping and whatever else. But with everything in the world causing cancer now, maybe they just see it differently than I do. Maybe they just aren't as scared of these things as I am. My sisters are both very strong!

I love my mom so much. It makes me so happy to see her doing so well. It gives me so much faith and hope. My baby will grow up to know her granny and to love her granny. I am so grateful for that everyday. I wish there were more ways for me to show her. I hope she always knows how much she means to me and everyone else!

My mom and I discussed living wills and things of that nature today. She told me she never wants to live off of a machine nor a feeding tube or any type of artificial means of life. She doesn't want to live as a vegetable. I agree with her. If there is no hope for me and there's nothing left for the doctors to do and they've proved it, I want to be put out of my misery too. It scares me to say that. It scares me to think about it. The whole prospect of death scares me. But I don't want my family to suffer. I want my family to be able to move on and be able to enjoy their lives.

I hope my children and my husband always know what they mean to me and how very much I love them. I want Kortney to always know that I adore her. I may not have had the honor of giving birth to her, but in my heart she is mine. I love that beautiful young lady just like I gave birth to her myself. She made me a mom and I am so grateful to her for that. She always brings out the best in me. She is my first child and my best friend. Her mom told me once that she is very happy that Kortney has me in her life. I hope Kortney always knows she is very lucky to be loved by so many people. I love you Koko. I hope Rylee Jo knows she's my angel, my sweet baby girl. I felt her grow in my tummy and watched her grow in my living room. I love her so much words can't express how I feel about her. The love I feel for her overwhelms me. I love you baby Rj. Then there's Joe, I love him so much. I never thought I would find this kind of love. He is my hero, he is my heart. I love Joe. Now, I'm not sure why I went on about that. I guess I just wanted it on record in case they ever wondered about how I felt about them. Maybe I'm just being sentimental and mushy today. Either way, they'll know how I feel about them.

14

Physical & hormone therapy

My mom finished her radiation and then began her physical therapy. She did it twice a week for a couple of weeks. They told her to order a bracelet letting everyone know in the event of an emergency not to take blood pressure or give shots on that arm. She will never be able to lift anything over 5lbs with that arm. She can never wear jewelry on that arm/hand again. She has to wear gloves if she's washing dishes. She can't get too hot. She can't do too much without taking a break. She's very limited with her left arm. I thought it was very sad that she can never wear her wedding ring again. It made me sad because I know how important it is to her. She has just a simple, plain ring. But it's so beautiful on her finger and it means the world to her. However, as usual she was very positive about it. She said, "Becky, it's a small sacrifice." I do realize that. I just wish she didn't have to give up so much. After all she's gone through she deserves more.

On Mother's Day, I felt horrible because the present I ordered her hadn't come in yet. So she wouldn't get her present until it finally got here! But I knew she didn't mind. She was very understanding.

Mom finished up everything except her hormone therapy. She has to take a pill called Arimidex for the next 5 years. It decreases the chances of the cancer returning by 50%. They did not give her tamoxifen because it can cause uterine cancer and she still has her uterus. Arimidex can only be given to women who have gone through menopause. They did blood work to verify she is post menopausal. Its worst side effects are bone loss and hot flashes. She has to lift weights, not to build muscle, but to build her bones. She is also supposed to drink 1-2 six ounce glasses of wine per day. That helps not only the heart, but it will help stop osteoporosis too. But anymore than 1-2 glasses a day will actually speed up osteoporosis. She made the comment to me, "I guess I will become a wine drinking body builder!" Now all she has left is follow up visits and checkups. She is doing so great. She has to wear her sleeve from about the time she gets up until about 7pm everyday. The sleeve is tan and almost looks just like her skin. It helps keep her arm compressed. I think it might help the flow of the fluids. The compression also helps reduce swelling as long as nothing interrupts the flow of the fluid (such as gnats or mosquito bites, lifting something heavy, bumps or cuts, etc.). She said it doesn't bother her though. She's a good sport.

I think about cancer a lot now. I wonder is it something we all need to gear up for. It seems to get everyone. Some survive, some don't. But it seems that in some way or another it affects all of us. I have changed my life style. I eat better and workout at least 3 days a week. I'm terrified of the day the doctor tells me I too have cancer. I'm trying to prevent in the best ways I know how. But can we really prevent it? I mean it seems like every time you turn around there's another thing causing cancer. Life is so short and I know everyone says that. But it really is. I look at my two beautiful daughters and it scares me that someday they might get cancer. I don't want them to ever have to go through chemotherapy or any pain for that matter. I'm so scared for them. I find myself buying products with the pink ribbon on them because I know some of the proceeds go to the cancer foundation. It means so much to me to help out in some way. I wish I could give more, but that's not always possible. I wish I could understand cancer. I read about it and research it. But I can't really understand it. I don't understand why it has to happen. I don't understand why it exist at all.

15

No more wig

My mom has stopped wearing her wig. Her hair is really short and it has lots of gray. They first day I saw her without it I was surprised. Not that it looked bad. I've just never seen my mom with gray hair. It floored me. Then I didn't know if I should tell her it looks nice or not bring attention to it. I know some people don't want to draw attention, but others want you to notice and open up about it. It didn't look bad at all. It looked very comfortable and relaxing. I do like my mom's hair better with color, probably because it's all I've ever know. I've never been a fan of gray hair, well not until you're about 70. Haha! Some people look very elegant and beautiful with gray hair. So I'm not trying to down anyone with gray hair, to each his own. I'm just saying, I'm not ready for it and do plan to dye my hair for sometime after it starts turning gray. My mom has always been that way too. I really didn't even know what the true color of my mom's hair is because for as long as I can remember she's dyed it. But it has always looked natural and beautiful. Even if she decides to keep the gray, she's still just as beautiful. It was just something I had never seen on her and it took me by surprise. Now it doesn't phase me at all. But I do hope that she didn't sense my astonishment when I saw her for the first time without her wig. Because I don't want to hurt her feelings. I just hope she knows I am so proud of her and so happy she finally got to take her wig off. I'm sure it was itchy and hot. She seemed so happy to have it off and I'm just as happy for her.

I met a man the other day that had cancer also. I felt so bad for him. He seemed so unhappy. He told me he never wished chemotherapy on his worst enemy. He told me he thought if he had to go through it just two more days it would have killed him. I just want to cry for him. I can't imagine what he must have gone through or what his family must have gone through. I just wanted to hold his hand and tell him to just keep the faith. I pray for him at night now too. I pray that this hasn't bent his soul forever. I know it may take time and I know it has to be hard. But I hope he's able to bridge his heart and soul back together and not let this destroy him. I knew him before the cancer and he was a funny, outgoing man. I pray he can get back to himself and so much more! He beat this, he is a survivor. I am so proud of him and his strength and courage to take on cancer and win!

I asked my mom today if she plans to dye her hair again when it grows out more. She said no, she thinks she'll let it go natural. I never thought I would say it, but I'm glad. I want her to be proud of herself and who she is and all that she stands for. She won her battle and not everyone gets the chance to say they beat cancer. She is an inspiration to millions and to me! My mom says she thinks she has found a side affect of the medicine she has to take for the next 5 years. She said she is very stiff now. She said sometimes it's painful. Getting out of bed is hard for her. She wanted so badly to bend down and hug my little girl the other day. It just proved to hard for her. But in the same notion she proclaimed she is still very grateful to be alive and that she could live with the stiffness. The courage and bravery in her heart and soul is never ending.

16

It's over

My mom is a survivor. My mom is a winner. As the daughter of a cancer survivor, I can never express how completely proud I am of my mom and all she has accomplished. But I can write a book about it and hope that she will always know and feel the love I have for her. She is the most beautiful, strong, intelligent woman I have ever had the honor and pleasure to know and love. With that I would like to leave the ending with a note to my mom:

Dearest Mom,

I want to thank you for all the years of my life and all the love you have given to me. You have been the best mom and role model ever! I can't imagine my life without you or our relationship. I will carry with me my whole life the values and morals you have taught me. I know how to dream and how to love with all my heart and how to be happy because of you. I know that life isn't always grand and that sometimes there are rainy days. But I also know that the sun will come out eventually. I know you get what you give and what comes around goes around. I know how to be true to myself and others. I know all of this because of you. You are my superwoman, my hero. My life has been truly happy and full of love and joy because you are in it. I love you so much and I will work to make sure you always feel that love.

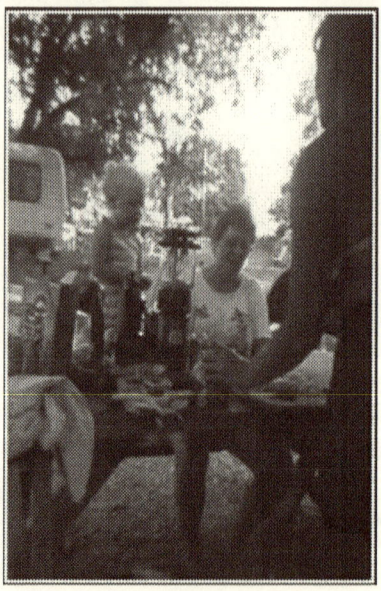

Love Always,
Becky

My beautiful mother, summer 2005………. cancer free!!!!

978-0-595-36527-2
0-595-36527-2

www.ingramcontent.com/pod-product-compliance
Lightning Source LLC
Chambersburg PA
CBHW050341290526
45785CB00006B/2585